Keto Slow Cooker Seafood Cookbook

50 easy and healthy Seafood Recipes for your keto slow cooker diet

Lilith Wolfe

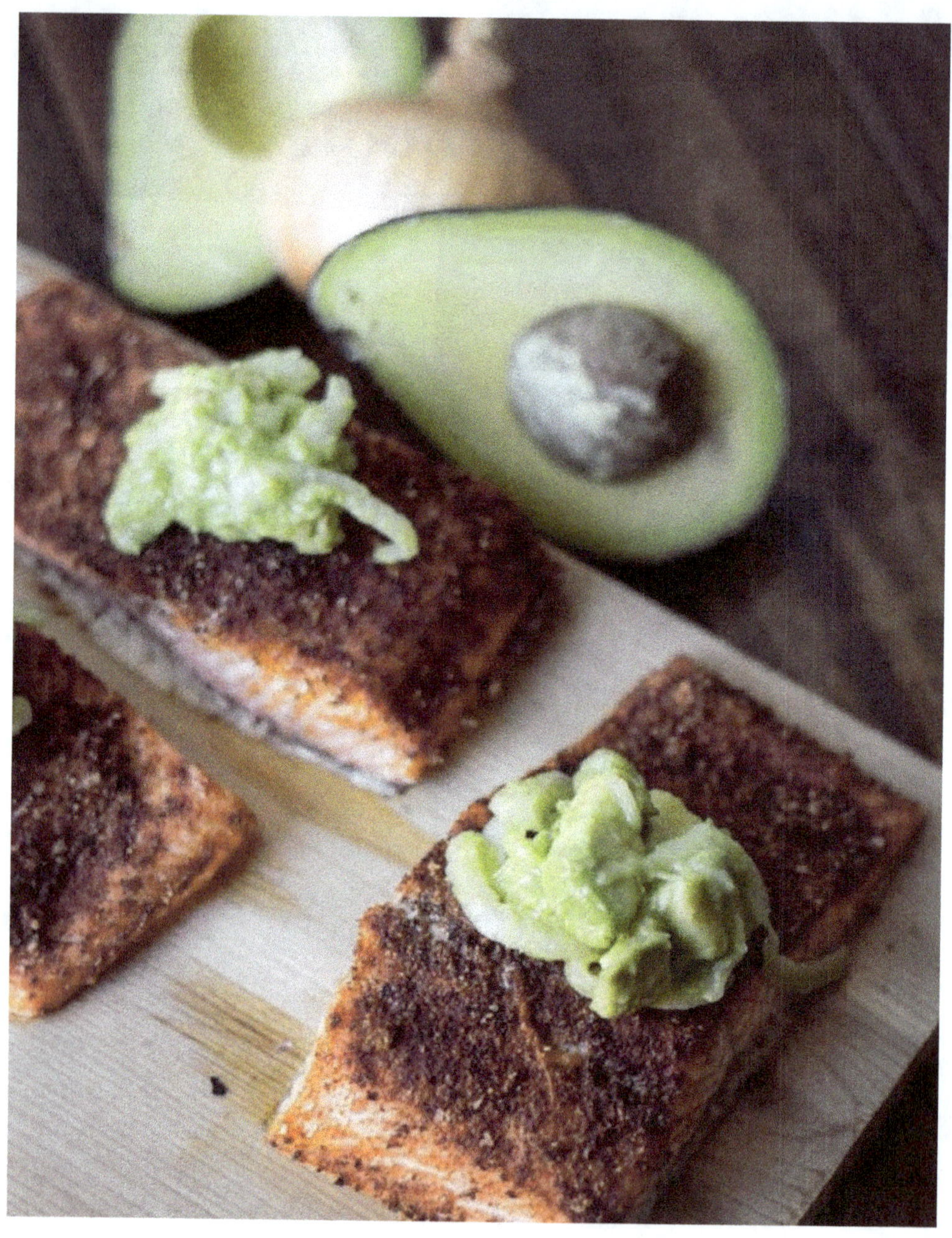

COPYRIGHT

Table of contents

Tilapia Filet

Preparation time: 15 minutes

Cooking time: 2 hours

Servings: 4

Ingredients:

4 tilapia fillets

For the garlic-butter compound:

8 tbsp. butter

8 chopped garlic cloves

8 tsp chopped parsley

Directions:

Mix all of the garlic-butter compound **Ingredients** in a mixing bowl.

Place each tilapia fillet in the middle of a large sheet of aluminum foil. Generously season fillets with salt and pepper.

Divide the garlic butter compound into each fillet, then seal all the fish's sides using a foil. Place into the slow cooker. Cover with lid—Cook for 2 hours on high.

Nutrition:

Calories: 309 Fat: 24.1 g

Protein: 21.9 g Carbs: 2.5 g

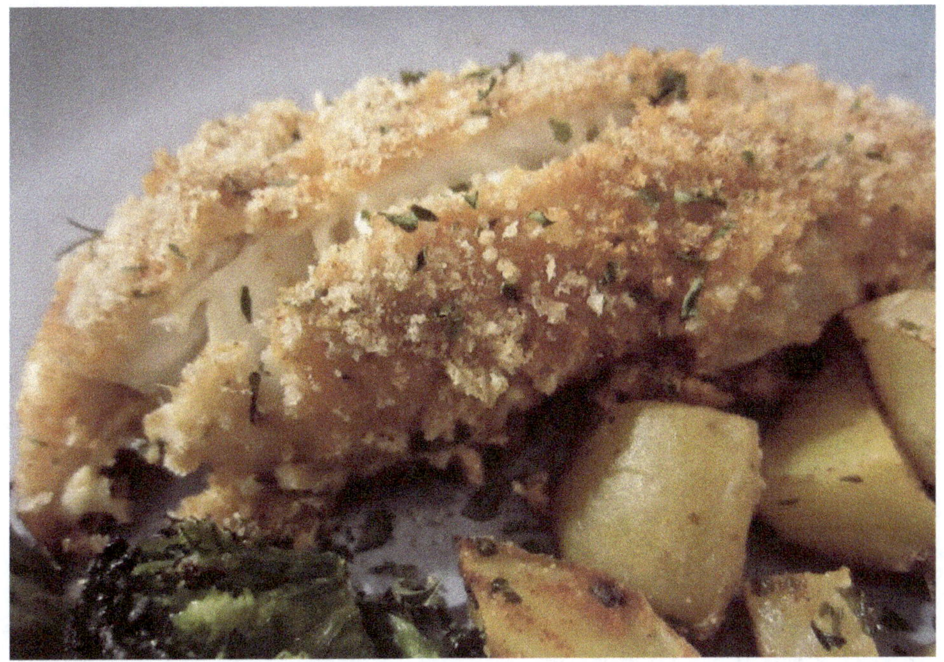

Tuna and Olive

Preparation time: 15 minutes

Cooking time: 1 hour

Servings: 4

Ingredients:

12 oz. tuna

5oz. pitted brine-cured black olives

5oz. pitted mild green olives

5 tbsps. extra-virgin olive oil, and extra for the spinach

6oz. fresh baby spinach

3 fresh bay leaves

2 thinly sliced garlic cloves

¼ c. fish stock or vegetable broth

¼ c. dry white or rose wine

½ tsp. kosher salt

½ medium finely chopped onion

1 tsp. red or white wine vinegar

1 orange zest

Directions:

In the slow cooker, combine the broth, wine, the 4 tablespoons olive oil, bay leaves, and salt. Season with pepper to taste. Stir to combine. Cover the slow cooker with lid. Cook for 30 minutes on low.

Add in the tuna. Turn to coat each piece evenly with the cooked broth wine mix. Cover and cook for 25-35 minutes on low or until the fish is opaque. When the fish is opaque, remove with a slotted spoon and transfer to a serving platter. Shred the fish into large flakes. Cover with foil to keep warm. Discard the cooking liquid.

While the fish is cooking, put the orange zest, garlic, olives, vinegar, and the remaining 1 tablespoon olive oil in a food processor. Pulse until the mix is a thick puree.

When ready to serve, put the spinach in a mixing bowl. Toss with a little olive oil—season with salt and pepper. Divide into the number of **Servings** indicated, creating a bed for the tuna. Evenly distribute the tuna flakes into the number of **Servings**. Top with the tapenade. Serve at room temperature.

Nutrition:

Calories: 414 Fat: 31 g

Protein: 25.1 g

Tuna Stuffed Mushroom

Preparation time: 15 minutes

Cooking time: 5 hours

Servings: 15

Ingredients:

8 oz. shredded Italian cheese blend

3 tbsp. mayonnaise

3 sliced scallions

3 oz. softened cream cheese

2 lbs. cleaned mushrooms

¼ c. minced fresh parsley

½ tsp. pepper

7 oz. drained tuna

14 oz drained chopped artichoke hearts

¼ tsp. hot sauce

Directions:

Place artichoke hearts, scallions, and the tuna in a mixing bowl and heat until well combined.

Then add in the Italian cheese, cream cheese, pepper, hot sauce, mayo, and parsley. Mash all your **Ingredients** until well blended.

Stuff the tuna-artichoke mix into the mushroom caps.

Place a basket-type steamer in the slow cooker. Arrange a layer of the stuffed mushrooms on the basket steamer.

Take a piece of aluminum foil, then make holes in the foil using a fork. Fit the holed aluminum foil down the first layer of the stuffed mushrooms. Make a hole in the middle.

Arrange another layer of stuffed mushrooms on the foil. Do the process again to ensure that the mushrooms are well arranged. Close the lid—Cook for about 4-5 hours on low.

When cooked, serve in the slow cooker to keep warm or transfer them into a serving platter.

Nutrition:

Calories: 142

Fat: 9 g

Protein: 10.7 g

Etouffee and olive

Preparation time: 15 minutes

Cooking time: 7 hours

Servings: 9

Ingredients:

1½ lbs. peeled and deveined raw shrimp

1½ lbs. quartered scallops

4 tbsp. olive oil

2 medium onions diced

9 scallions, chopped

3 celery stalks, diced

2 diced small green bell peppers

2 diced small jalapeno peppers

3 minced garlic cloves

20oz. diced tomatoes

5 tbsp tomato paste

¾ tsp dried basil

¾ tsp dried thyme

¾ tsp dried oregano

1/3 tsp cayenne pepper

3 tsp almond meal

1½ tbsp. cold water

Hot sauce

Sea salt

Directions:

Combine the olive oil and onion in the slow cooker. Add the scallions, bell pepper, jalapeno, and celery. Mix well.

Cook within 30 minutes, high.

Add the tomato paste and garlic—cover and cook for 15 minutes on high.

Add the tomatoes, cayenne, thyme, oregano, basil, and salt—Cook within 6 hours on low.

Add the shrimp and scallops. Set heat to high, cover, and cook for 15 minutes.

Combine the almond meal and water. Add the mixture in your slow cooker for about 6 minutes to thicken. Add a few drops of hot sauce and stir.

Nutrition:

Calories: 247

Protein: 19 g

Fat: 1.3 g

Carbs: 6.2 g

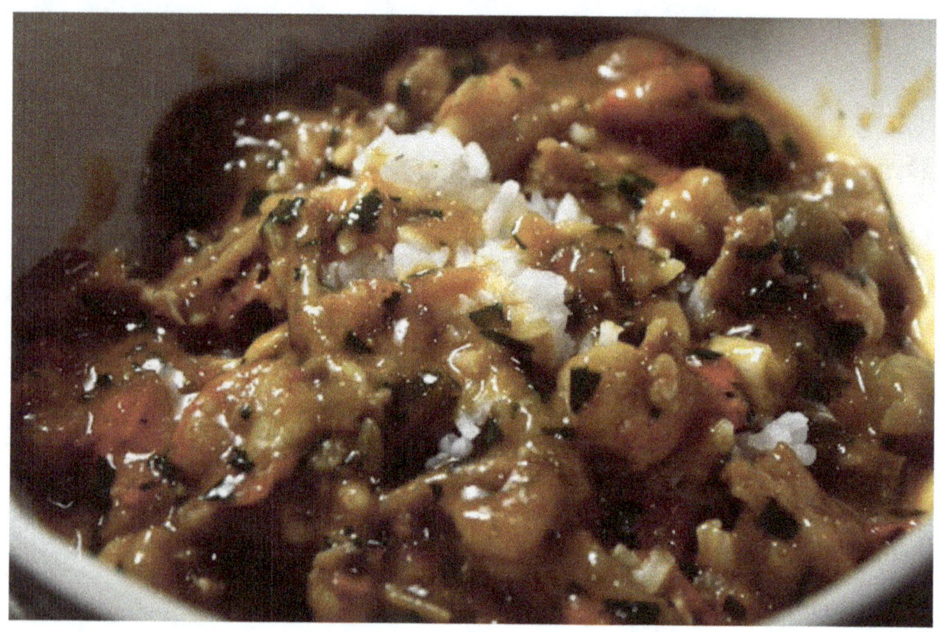

Salty Salmon

Preparation time: 15 minutes

Cooking time: 1 hour

Servings: 8

Ingredients:

2 tbsps. butter

1 sliced large sweet onion

3 c. water

2 tbsps. lemon juice

2 sprigs fresh dill

8 salmon fillets

Sea salt

2 quartered lemons

Directions:

Butter the inside of the slow cooker. Place the onion rings on the bottom in a single layer.

Slowly pour the water into the slow cooker—Cook within a half an hour on high.

On top of the onion slices, place salmon fillets—season with the fresh dill, salt, and some lemon juice.

Cover the cooker and cook for 30 mins on high or until the salmon is no longer pink on the outside.

Drain the fillets very well and serve with the lemon wedges.

Nutrition:

Calories: 100 Protein: 40.1 g

Fat: 3.4 g Carbs: 3.75 g

Fish Soup

Preparation time: 15 minutes

Cooking time: 4 hours

Servings: 3

Ingredients:

½ qt chicken broth

¼ c. dry red wine or chicken broth

1½ lb. chopped tomatoes

1 chopped medium onion

1½ minced garlic cloves garlic

½ tsp dried oregano

½ tsp dried sage

½ tsp. dried rosemary leaves

1/8 tsp. red pepper, crushed

¾ lb. assorted skinless fish fillets

3 oz. peeled and deveined shrimp

Salt

Pepper

3 slices Italian bread, toasted

1 halved clove garlic

Directions:

In a slow cooker, mix all of the **Ingredients** except the seafood, salt, pepper, bread, and halved garlic cloves. Cook on high for 4 hours.

In the last 15 minutes, add the seafood—season with salt and pepper.

In the meantime, rub the garlic cloves on the bread. Place bread into soup bowls and ladle the soup on top. Serve piping hot.

Nutrition:

Calories: 132.2 Fat: 3.3 g

Carbs: 18.9 g

Protein: 7.6 g

Hot Chili Shrimps

Preparation time: 15 minutes

Cooking time: 2 hours

Servings: 6

Ingredients:

1½ pounds peeled and deveined raw shrimps

1-pound tomatoes, fire-roasted

2 tablespoons spicy salsa

½ c. chopped bell pepper

Sea salt

Black pepper

½ teaspoon cumin

½ teaspoon cayenne pepper

½ teaspoon minced garlic

4 tablespoons chopped cilantro

2 tablespoons olive oil

Directions:

Drizzle the slow cooker with a generous amount of olive oil. Place the shrimps at the bottom of it.

Put the rest of the fixing into the slow cooker. Cook on high for 2 hours.

Nutrition:

Calories: 185 Fat: 6.7 g

Carbs: 5.2 g Protein: 28.4 g

Fennel Scented Fish Stew

Preparation time: 15 minutes

Cooking time: 6 hours

Servings: 4

Ingredients:

½ qt clam juice

¼ c. dry white wine

2½ peeled and chopped medium tomatoes

½ c. carrots, chopped

½ c. onion, chopped

1½ minced garlic cloves

½ tbsp minced orange zest

½ tsp. lightly crushed fennel seeds

1 lb. firm fish fillets, chopped

1/8 c. parsley chopped

Salt

Pepper

Directions:

In a slow cooker, mix all the **Ingredients**, except the fish fillets, parsley, salt, and pepper. Cook on low for 6 hours. Add the fish within the last 15 minutes. Add the parsley and stir to distribute—season with salt and pepper before serving.

Nutrition:

Calories: 342 Fat: 8.2 g

Carbs: 21 g Protein: 36 g

Chinese Oyster Soup

Preparation time: 15 minutes

Cooking time: 6 hours

Servings: 2

Ingredients:

1¼ c. chicken broth

1 tbsp. soy sauce

1 c. sliced Napa cabbage

4 o sliced mushrooms

½ tbsp. ginger root, minced

½ pint fresh oysters

Salt

Pepper

Directions:

In a slow cooker, mix the broth, soy sauce, cabbage, mushrooms, bean sprouts, green onions, and ginger root. Cook for 6 hours on low. In the last 15 minutes, put the oysters and liquid—season with salt and pepper before serving.

Nutrition:

Calories: 206.89 Fat: 5.93 g

Carbs: 5.1 g Protein: 30.98 g

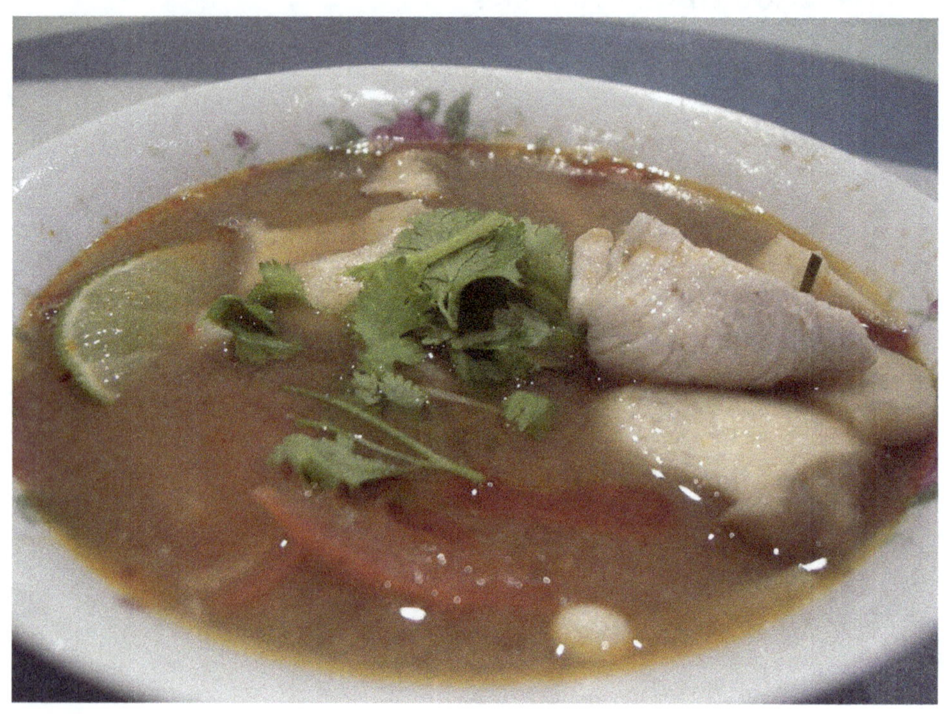

Hearty White Fish Stew

Preparation time: 15 minutes

Cooking time: 6 hours

Servings: 3

Ingredients:

1½ pounds sliced white fish

2 tbsps. butter

1-pound diced tomatoes

2 small sliced zucchinis

1 minced clove garlic

1 chopped large onion

1 chopped green bell pepper

½ teaspoon basil, dried

½ teaspoon oregano, dried

Salt

Black pepper

¼ c. fish stock

Directions:

Stir in everything together in the slow cooker pot. Put and secure the lid. Cook the dish on high for 5-6 hours. Serve.

Nutrition:

Calories: 168

Fat: 6.8 g

Carbs: 4.5 g

Protein: 16.4 g

Catfish Creole

Preparation time: 15 minutes

Cooking time: 4 hours

Servings: 3

Ingredients:

8 oz. diced tomatoes

¼ c. clam juice or chicken broth

1½ tbsp tomato paste

¼ c. medium onion, chopped

¼ c. green bell pepper, chopped

2 sliced green onions

½ thinly sliced rib celery

2 minced garlic cloves

¼ tsp dried marjoram and thyme leaves

½ tsp celery seeds

½ tsp. ground cumin

¾ lb. catfish fillets

Sal t

Hot pepper sauce

Red Pepper Rice:

¾ c. uncooked long-grain rice

1/8tsp. ground turmeric

¼ tsp. paprika

½ coarsely chopped roasted red pepper

Directions:

Mix all of the catfish creole **Ingredients**, except the catfish fillets, salt, and red pepper sauce, in the slow cooker. Cook on high for 4 hours.

Add the fish within the last 15 minutes—season with salt and hot pepper sauce. Serve with Red Pepper Rice.

To make Red Pepper Rice, cook the long grain rice-based on package instructions. Add the turmeric into the cooking water.

After the rice is cooked, add the paprika and roasted red pepper and stir gently to distribute.

Nutrition:

Calories: 580

Fat: 5 g

Carbs: 26 g

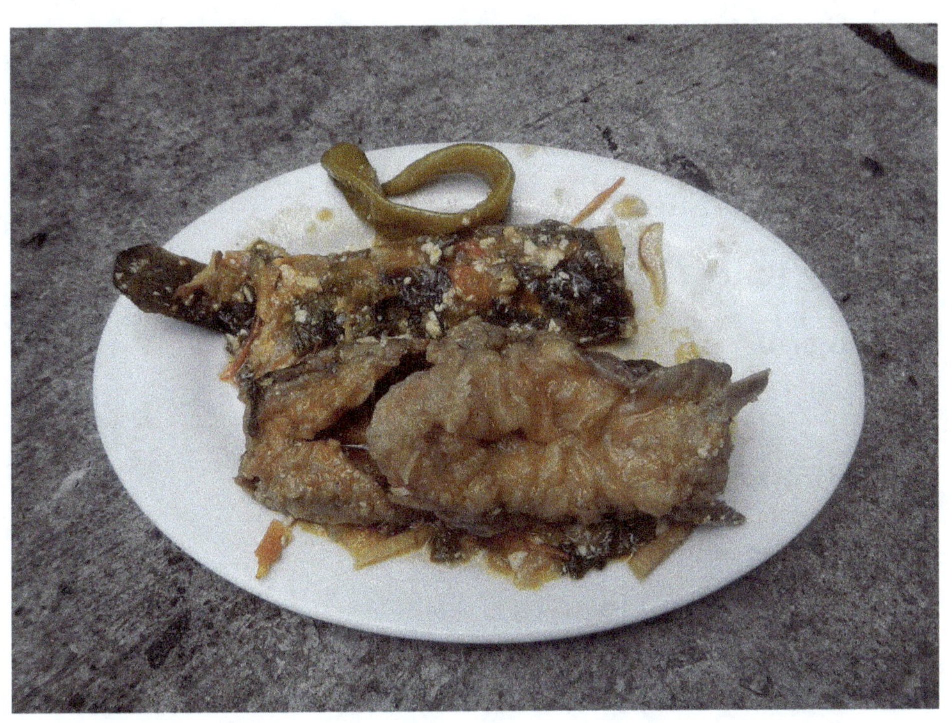

Mexican Corn and Shrimp Soup

Preparation time: 15 minutes

Cooking time: 4 hours & 10 minutes

Servings: 2

Ingredients:

1 c. reduced-sodium vegetable broth

2½ c. whole kernel corn

1/3 c. onion, chopped

1 small jalapeno chili, minced

1 minced garlic clove

1 tbsp. chopped epazote leaves

6 oz. peeled and deveined shrimp

Salt

Cayenne pepper

Roasted Red Pepper Sauce:

1 halved large red bell pepper

½ tsp. sugar

Directions:

In a slow cooker, mix all the **Ingredients**, except the epazote, shrimp, salt, and cayenne pepper. Cook on high for 4 hours.

Blend the soup into a food processor or blender and add the epazote leaves. Blend until smooth and pour back into a slow cooker. Add the shrimp. Cook within 10 minutes on high. Season with salt and pepper.

To make the Roasted Red Pepper Sauce, put the pepper with the skin side up on a broiler pan. Broil until the skin becomes blackened and blistered.

Transfer the roasted pepper into a plastic bag and set aside for 5 minutes. Then, peel off the skin. Blend with the sugar in a food processor or blender until smooth.

Soup can be served warm or chilled. Add 3 tablespoons of Roasted Red Pepper Sauce into each serving bowl.

Nutrition:

Calories: 194.9

Carbs: 24.2 g

Fat: 6.3 g

Protein: 13.6 g

Cod with Fennel and Tomatoes

Preparation time: 15 minutes

Cooking time: 7 hours & 45 minutes

Servings: 8

Ingredients:

4 medium fennel bulbs, stalks discarded

½ c. olive oil

2 large sliced onions

4 minced cloves garlic

48 ounces diced tomatoes

1 c. white wine, dry

2 tablespoons lemon zest, grated

1 c. lemon juice

2 tablespoons fennel seeds, crushed

4 pounds cod fillets

Sea salt

Black pepper

Directions:

Rinse the fennel, then remove the core and outermost flesh. Slice thinly and set aside.

Place a skillet over a medium-high flame and heat the oil. Sauté the onion and garlic until onion becomes translucent. Stir in the fennel and cook for 2 minutes. Transfer into the slow cooker.

Stir the tomatoes, lemon zest and juice, wine, and fennel seeds into the slow cooker—Cook within 7 hours on low. Season the fish with salt and pepper.

Increase heat to high and add the fish into the slow cooker. Cook within 45 minutes or until the fish is cooked through.

Nutrition:

Calories: 217

Carbs: 12.9 g

Protein: 41.4 g

Fat: 29.1 g

Mahi-Mahi Taco Wraps

Preparation time: 5 minutes

Cooking time: 2 hours

Servings: 6

Ingredients:

1-pound Mahi-Mahi, wild-caught

½ cup cherry tomatoes

1 green bell pepper

1/4 medium red onion

½ teaspoon garlic powder

1 teaspoon of sea salt

½ teaspoon ground black pepper

1 teaspoon chipotle pepper

½ teaspoon dried oregano

1 teaspoon cumin

2 tablespoons avocado oil

1/4 cup chicken stock

1 medium avocado, diced

1 cup sour cream

6 large lettuce leaves

Directions:

Grease a 6-quarts slow cooker with oil, place fish in it and then pour in chicken stock.

Stir together garlic powder, salt, black pepper, chipotle pepper, oregano, and cumin and then season fish with half of this mixture.

Layer fish with tomatoes, pepper, and onion, season with remaining spice mixture, and shut with lid.

Plugin the slow cooker, then cook fish for 2 hours at a high heat setting or until cooked.

When done, evenly spoon fish among lettuce, top with avocado and sour cream, and serve.

Nutrition:

Calories: 193.6

Fat: 12g

Protein: 17g

Carbs: 5g

Fiber: 3g

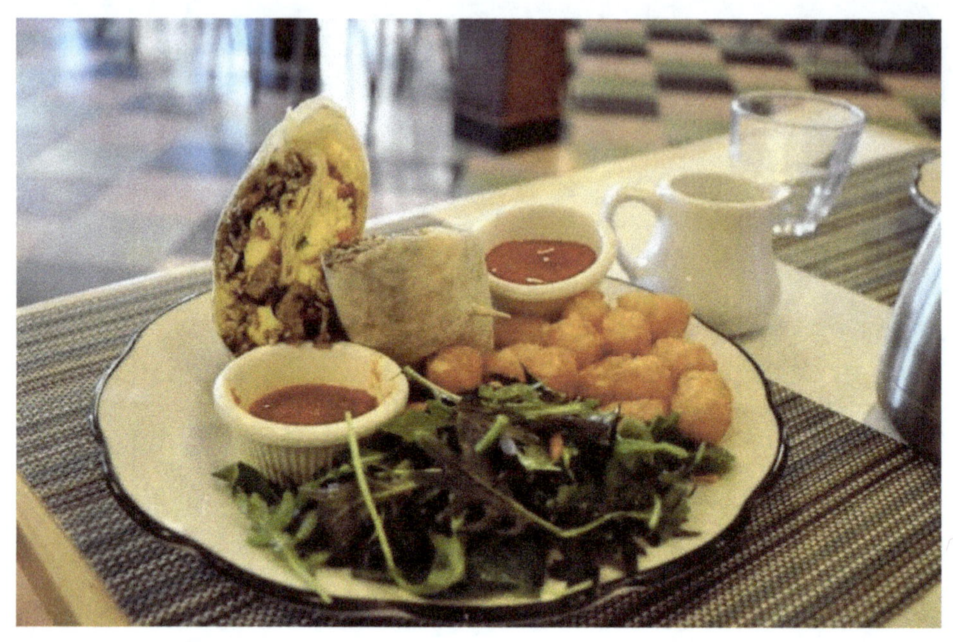

Shrimp Scampi

Preparation time: 5 minutes

Cooking time: 2 hours & 30 minutes

Servings: 4

Ingredients:

1 pound wild-caught shrimps, peeled & deveined

1 tablespoon minced garlic

1 teaspoon salt

½ teaspoon ground black pepper

1/2 teaspoon red pepper flakes

2 tablespoons chopped parsley

2 tablespoons avocado oil

2 tablespoons unsalted butter

1/2 cup white wine

1 tablespoon lemon juice

1/4 cup chicken broth

½ cup grated parmesan cheese

Directions:

Place all the **Ingredients** except for shrimps and cheese in a 6-quart slow cooker and whisk until combined. Add shrimps and stir until evenly coated and shut with lid. Cook in the slow cooker for 1 hour and 30 minutes to 2 hours and 30 minutes at low heat setting or until cooked. Then top with parmesan cheese and serve.

Nutrition:

Calories: 234 Total Fat: 14.7g Protein: 23.3g

Carbs: 2.1g Fiber: 0.1g Sugar: 2g

Shrimp Tacos

Preparation time: 5 minutes

Cooking time: 3 hours

Servings: 6

Ingredients:

1 pound medium wild-caught shrimp, peeled and tails off

12-ounce fire-roasted tomatoes, diced

1 small green bell pepper, chopped

½ cup chopped white onion

1 teaspoon minced garlic

½ teaspoon of sea salt

½ teaspoon ground black pepper

½ teaspoon red chili powder

½ teaspoon cumin

¼ teaspoon cayenne pepper

2 tablespoons avocado oil

1/2 cup salsa

4 tablespoons chopped cilantro

1 ½ cup sour cream

2 medium avocados, diced

Directions:

Rinse shrimps, layer into a 6-quarts slow cooker, and drizzle with oil.

Add tomatoes, stir until mixed, then add peppers and remaining **Ingredients** except for sour cream and avocado and stir until combined.

Plugin the slow cooker, shut with lid, and cook for 2 to 3 hours at low heat setting or 1 hour and 30 minutes to 2 hours at high heat setting or until shrimps turn pink.

When done, serve shrimps with avocado and sour cream.

Nutrition:

Calories: 369

Fat: 27.5g

Protein: 21.2g

Carbs: 9.2g

Fiber: 5g

Sugar: 5g

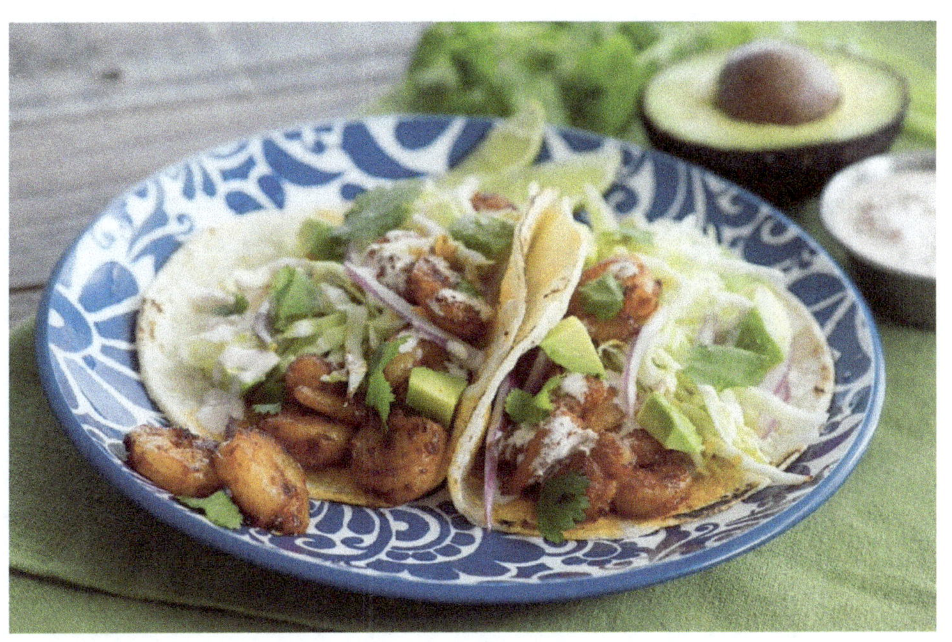

Fish Curry

Preparation time: 5 minutes

Cooking time: 4 hours 7 30 minutes

Servings: 6

Ingredients:

2.2 pounds wild-caught white fish fillet, cubed

18-ounce spinach leaves

4 tablespoons red curry paste, organic

14-ounce coconut cream, unsweetened and full-fat

14-ounce water

Directions:

Plug in a 6-quart slow cooker and let preheat at high heat setting.

In the meantime, whisk together coconut cream and water until smooth.

Place fish into the slow cooker, spread with curry paste, and then pour in coconut cream mixture.

Cook within 2 hours at a high setting or 4 hours at low heat setting until tender.

Then add spinach and continue cooking for 20 to 30 minutes or until spinach leaves wilt.

Serve straight away.

Nutrition:

Calories: 323

Fat: 51.5g

Protein: 41.3g

Carbs: 7g

Fiber: 2.2g

Sugar: 2.3g

Salmon with Creamy Lemon Sauce

Preparation time: 5 minutes

Cooking time: 2 hours & 15 minutes

Servings: 6

Ingredients:

For the Salmon:

2 pounds wild-caught salmon fillet, skin-on

1 teaspoon garlic powder

1 ½ teaspoon salt

1 teaspoon ground black pepper

1/2 teaspoon red chili powder

1 teaspoon Italian Seasoning

1 lemon, sliced

1 lemon, juiced

2 tablespoons avocado oil

1 cup chicken broth

For the Creamy Lemon Sauce:

Chopped parsley, for garnish

1/8 teaspoon lemon zest

1/4 cup heavy cream

1/4 cup grated parmesan cheese

Directions:

Line a 6-quart slow cooker with parchment sheet spread its bottom with lemon slices, top with salmon and drizzle with oil.

Stir together garlic powder, salt, black pepper, red chili powder, Italian seasoning, and oil until combined and rub this mixture all over salmon.

Pour lemon juice and broth around the fish and shut with lid.

Cook in the slow cooker within 2 hours at a low heat setting.

In the meantime, set the oven at 400 degrees F and let preheat.

When fish is done, lift out an inner pot of slow cooker, place into the oven, then cook within 5 to 8 minutes or until the top is nicely browned.

Lift out the fish using a parchment sheet and keep it warm.

Remove, transfer juices to a medium skillet pan, place it over medium-high heat, and then bring to boil and cook for 1 minute.

Turn heat to a low level, whisk the cream into the sauce, and lemon zest and parmesan cheese and cook for 2 to 3 minutes or until thickened.

Cut salmon in pieces, then top each portion with lemon sauce and serve.

Nutrition:

Calories: 340

Fat: 20g

Protein: 32g

Carbs: 8g

Fiber: 2g

Salmon with Lemon-Caper Sauce

Preparation time: 5 minutes

Cooking time: 1 hour & 30 minutes

Servings: 6

Ingredients:

1 pound wild-caught salmon fillet

2 teaspoon capers, rinsed and mashed

1 teaspoon minced garlic

1 teaspoon salt

½ teaspoon ground black pepper

1/2 teaspoon dried oregano

1 teaspoon lemon zest

2 tablespoons lemon juice

4 tablespoons unsalted butter

Directions:

Cut salmon into 4 pieces, then season with salt and black pepper and sprinkle lemon zest on top.

Arrange a 6-quart slow cooker with parchment paper, place seasoned salmon pieces on it, and shut with lid.

Set to cook in the slow cooker within 1 hour and 30 minutes or until salmon is cooked through. Prepare lemon-caper sauce and for this, place a small saucepan over low heat, add butter and let it melt. Then add capers, garlic, lemon juice, stir until mixed and simmer for 1 minute.

Remove saucepan from heat and stir in oregano. When salmon is cooked, spoon lemon-caper sauce on it and serve.

Nutrition:

Calories: 368.5 Fat: 26.6g

Protein: 19.5g Carbs: 2.7g

Fiber: 0.3g Sugar: 2g

Spicy Barbecue Shrimp

Preparation time: 5 minutes

Cooking time: 1 hour & 30 minutes

Servings: 6

Ingredients:

1 1/2 pounds large wild-caught shrimp, unpeeled

1 green onion, chopped

1 teaspoon minced garlic

1 ½ teaspoon salt

¾ teaspoon ground black pepper

1 teaspoon Cajun seasoning

1 tablespoon hot pepper sauce

¼ cup Worcestershire Sauce

1 lemon, juiced

2 tablespoons avocado oil

1/2 cup unsalted butter, chopped

Directions:

Place all the **Ingredients** except for shrimps in a 6-quart slow cooker and whisk until mixed.

Plugin the slow cooker, then shut with lid and cook for 1 hour and 30 minutes at a high heat setting.

Then take out ½ cup of this sauce and reserve.

Add shrimps to slow cooker.

Nutrition:

Calories: 321

Fat: 21.4g

Protein: 27.3g

Carbs: 4.8g

Fiber: 2.4g

Sugar: 1.2g

Lemon Dill Halibut

Preparation time: 15 minutes

Cooking time: 2 hours

Servings: 2

Ingredients:

12-ounce wild-caught halibut fillet

1 teaspoon salt

½ teaspoon ground black pepper

1 1/2 teaspoon dried dill

1 tablespoon fresh lemon juice

3 tablespoons avocado oil

Directions:

Cut an 18-inch piece of aluminum foil, halibut fillet in the middle, and then season with salt and black pepper.

Whisk the remaining **Ingredients**, drizzle this mixture over halibut, then crimp foil's edges and place it into a 6-quart slow cooker.

Cook within 1 hour and 30 minutes or 2 hours at high heat setting or until cooked.

When done, carefully open the crimped edges and check the fish; it should be tender and flaky.

Serve straight away.

Nutrition:

Calories: 321.5 Fat: 21.4g

Protein: 32.1g Carbs: 0g

Fiber: 0g

Sugar: 0.6g

Coconut Cilantro Curry Shrimp

Preparation time: 15 minutes

Cooking time: 2 hours & 30 minutes

Servings: 4

Ingredients:

1 pound wild-caught shrimp, peeled and deveined

2 ½ teaspoon lemon garlic seasoning

2 tablespoons red curry paste

4 tablespoons chopped cilantro

30 ounces coconut milk, unsweetened

16 ounces of water

Directions:

Whisk together all the **Ingredients** except for shrimps and 2 tablespoons cilantro and add to a 4-quart slow cooker.

Plugin the slow cooker, shut with lid, and cook for 2 hours at high heat setting or 4 hours at low heat setting.

Then add shrimps, toss until evenly coated and cook for 20 to 30 minutes at high heat settings or until shrimps are pink.

Garnish shrimps with remaining cilantro and serve.

Nutrition:

Calories: 160.7 Total Fat: 8.2g

Protein: 19.3g

Carbs: 2.4g

Fiber: 0.5g

Sugar: 1.4g

Shrimp in Marinara Sauce

Preparation time: 15 minutes

Cooking time:5 hours & 10 minutes

Servings: 5

Ingredients:

1 pound cooked wild-caught shrimps, peeled and deveined

14.5-ounce crushed tomatoes

½ teaspoon minced garlic

1 teaspoon salt

1/2 teaspoon seasoned salt

¼ teaspoon ground black pepper

½ teaspoon crushed red pepper flakes

1/2 teaspoon dried basil

1/2 teaspoon dried oregano

½ tablespoons avocado oil

6-ounce chicken broth

2 tablespoon minced parsley

1/2 cup grated Parmesan cheese

Directions:

Place all the **Ingredients** except for shrimps, parsley, and cheese in a 4-quart slow cooker and stir well.

Then plug in the slow cooker, shut with lid, and cook for 4 to 5 hours at a low heat setting.

Then add shrimps and parsley, stir until mixed and cook for 10 minutes at high heat setting.

Garnish shrimps with cheese and serve.

Nutrition:

Calories: 358.8

Fat: 25.1g

Protein: 26g

Carbs: 7.2g

Fiber: 1.5g

Sugar: 3.6g

Garlic Shrimp

Preparation time: 5 minutes

Cooking time: 1 hour

Servings: 5

Ingredients:

For the Garlic Shrimp:

1 1/2 pounds large wild-caught shrimp, peeled and deveined

1/4 teaspoon ground black pepper

1/8 teaspoon ground cayenne pepper

2 ½ teaspoons minced garlic

1/4 cup avocado oil

4 tablespoons unsalted butter

For the Seasoning:

1 teaspoon onion powder

1 tablespoon garlic powder

1 tablespoon salt

2 teaspoons ground black pepper

1 tablespoon paprika

1 teaspoon cayenne pepper

1 teaspoon dried oregano

1 teaspoon dried thyme

Directions:

Stir together all the **Ingredients** for seasoning, garlic, oil, and butter and add to a 4-quart slow cooker.

Plugin the slow cooker, shut with lid, and cook for 25 to 30 minutes at high heat setting or until cooked.

Then add shrimps, toss until evenly coated, and continue cooking for 20 to 30 minutes at high heat setting or until shrimps are pink.

When done, transfer shrimps to a serving plate, top with sauce, and serve.

Nutrition:

Calories: 233.6

Fat: 11.7g

Protein: 30.9g

Carbs: 1.2g

Fiber: 0g

Sugar: 0 g

Lemon Pepper Tilapia

Preparation time: 5 minutes

Cooking time: 3 hours

Servings: 6

Ingredients:

6 wild-caught Tilapia fillets

4 teaspoons lemon-pepper seasoning, divided

6 tablespoons unsalted butter, divided

1/2 cup lemon juice, fresh

Directions:

Put each fillet in the center of the foil, then season with lemon-pepper seasoning, drizzle with lemon juice, and top with 1 tablespoon butter.

Gently crimp the edges of foil to form a packet and place it into a 6-quart slow cooker.

Plugin the slow cooker, shut with lid, and cook for 3 hours at high heat or until cooked.

Serve straight away.

Nutrition:

Calories: 201.2

Fat: 12.9g

Protein: 19.6g

Carbs: 1.5g

Fiber: 0.3g

Sugar: 0.7g

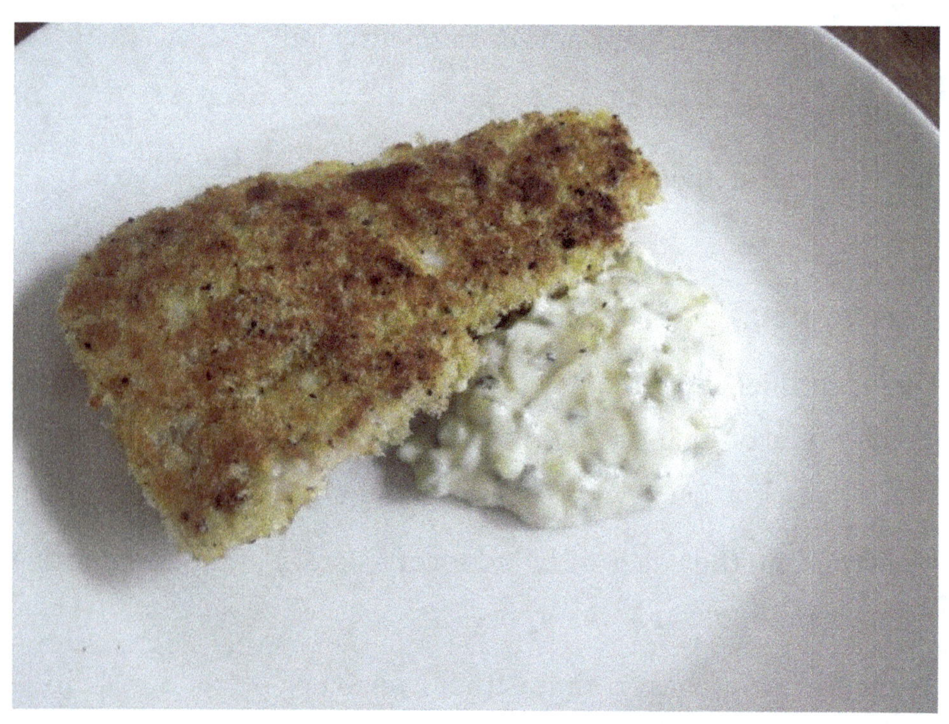

Clam Chowder

Preparation time: 15 minutes

Cooking time: 6 hours

Servings: 6

Ingredients:

20-ounce wild-caught baby clams, with juice

½ cup chopped scallion

½ cup chopped celery

1 teaspoon salt

1 teaspoon ground black pepper

1 teaspoon dried thyme

1 tablespoon avocado oil

2 cups coconut cream, full-fat

2 cups chicken broth

Directions:

Grease a 6-quart slow cooker with oil, then add **Ingredients** and stir until mixed.

Plugin the slow cooker, shut with lid, and cook for 4 to 6 hours at low heat setting or until cooked.

Serve straight away.

Nutrition:

Calories: 357 Fat: 28.9g

Protein: 15.2g Carbs: 8.9g

Fiber: 2.1g Sugar: 3.9g

Soy-Ginger Steamed Pompano

Preparation time: 5 minutes

Cooking time: 1 hour

Servings: 4

Ingredients:

1 wild-caught whole pompano, gutted and scaled

1 bunch scallion, diced

1 bunch cilantro, chopped

3 teaspoons minced garlic

1 tablespoon grated ginger

1 tablespoon swerve sweetener

¼ cup of soy sauce

¼ cup white wine

¼ cup sesame oil

Directions:

Place scallions in a 6-quart slow cooker and top with fish.

Whisk together remaining **Ingredients**, except for cilantro, and pour the mixture all over the fish.

Plugin the slow cooker, shut with lid, and cook for 1 hour at high heat or until cooked.

Garnish with cilantro and serve.

Nutrition:

Calories: 202.5 Fat: 24.2g

Protein: 22.7g Carbs: 4g

Fiber: 0.5g Sugar: 1.1g

Vietnamese Braised Catfish

Preparation time: 5 minutes

Cooking time: 6 hours

Servings: 3

Ingredients:

1 fillet of wild-caught catfish, cut into bite-size pieces

1 scallion, chopped

3 red chilies, chopped

1 tablespoon grated ginger

1/2 cup swerve sweetener

2 tablespoons avocado oil

1/4 cup fish sauce, unsweetened

Directions:

Put a small saucepan over medium heat, put the sweetener, and cook until it melts.

Then add scallion, chilies, ginger, and fish sauce and stir until mixed.

Transfer this mixture in a 4-quart slow cooker, add fish and toss until coated.

Plugin the slow cooker, shut with lid, and cook for 6 hours at low heat setting until cooked.

Drizzle with avocado oil and serve straight away.

Nutrition:

Calories: 110.7 Fat: 8g Protein: 9.4g

Carbs: 0.3g Fiber: 0.2g

Poached Salmon in Court-Bouillon Recipe

Preparation time: 5 minutes

Cooking time: 2 hours 30 minutes

Servings: 2

Ingredients:

2 whole black peppercorns

1/2 medium carrot, thinly sliced

1/2 celery rib, thinly sliced

2 salmon steaks in 1-inch-thick slice s

1 1/2 tbsp white wine vinegar

Directions:

Put all the items in the crockpot except for the salmon. You can also add parsley and bay leaf for extra flavor. Rub salmon slices with salt and pepper to taste. Cook within 2 hours on high.

Put some of the liquid over the top. Cook again within 30 minutes, high.

Nutrition:

Calories: 197 Fat: 7.7g Carbs: 4.8g

Protein: 18.3g Cholesterol: 95mg

Sodium: 366mg

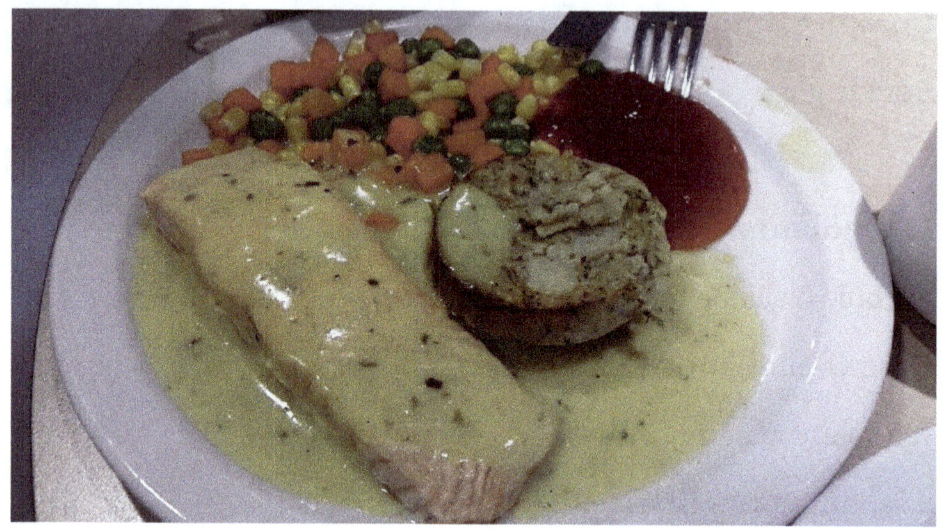

Braised Squid with Tomatoes and Fennel

Preparation time: 20 minutes

Cooking time: 4 hours

Servings: 2

Ingredients:

1 1/2 cups clam juice

1 can plum tomatoes

1/2 fennel bulb, minced

3 tbsp all-purpose flour

1 lb. squid in 1-inch pieces

Directions:

Add chopped onions, fennel, and garlic to the flameproof insert of a crockpot and cook on a stove in medium heat for about 5 minutes.

Whisk in flour and tomato paste until thoroughly mixed, then add the clam juice, tomatoes, 1 tsp salt, and pepper. Boil for about 2 minutes.

Transfer to the crockpot, cover, and cook for 3 hours on low.

Uncover, add the squid and mix well—Cook for another 1 hour.

Nutrition:

Calories: 210

Fat: 25g

Carbs: 6g

Protein: 29g

Seafood Stir-Fry Soup

Preparation time: 30 minutes

Cooking time: 3 hours & 10 minutes

Servings: 2

Ingredients:

7.25 oz low-carb Udon noodle, beef flavor

1/2 lb. shrimp

1/4 lb. scallops

3 cups low-sodium broth

1 carrot, shredded

Directions:

Add all **Ingredients** except noodles, shrimp, and scallops to the crockpot. Include seasonings such as garlic, ginger, salt, and pepper to taste. Add vinegar, soy sauce, and fish sauce, 1/2 tbsp each. Stir to mix well.

Cook on high for 2-3 hours. Add udon noodles, shrimp, and scallops. Cook on high for additional 10-15 minutes.

Nutrition:

Calories: 266

Fat: 19g

Carbs: 8g

Protein: 27.5g

Cholesterol: 173mg

Sodium: 489mg

Shrimp Fajita Soup

Preparation time: 20 minutes

Cooking time: 2 hours

Servings: 2

Ingredients:

1/2 lb. shrimp

32 oz chicken broth

1 tbsp fajita seasoning

1/2 bell pepper, sliced or diced

Directions:

Put all the listed items except the shrimp in the crockpot. Add onion slices to taste and stir to mix well.

Cook on high for 2 hours. Add the shrimp, and cook for additional 5-15 minutes.

Nutrition:

Calories: 165

Fat: 7.3g

Carbs: 3.7g

Protein: 15.9g

Cholesterol: 87mg

Sodium: 215mg

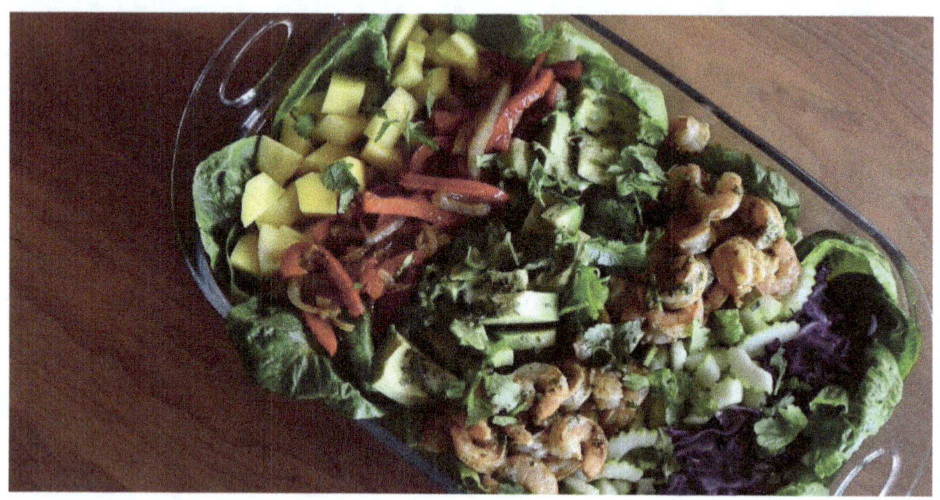

Fish and Tomatoes

Preparation time: 7 minutes

Cooking time: 3 hours

Servings: 2

Ingredients:

1/2 bell pepper, sliced

1/8 cup low-sodium broth

8 oz diced tomatoes

1/2 tbsp rosemary

1/2 lb. cod

Directions:

Put all the listed fixing except the fish in the crockpot. Add garlic, salt, and pepper to taste.

Season fish with your favorite seasoning and place other **Ingredients** in the pot. Cook for 3 hours on low.

Nutrition:

Calories: 204 Fat: 16.8g

Carbs: 5g Protein: 25.3g

Cholesterol: 75mg Sodium: 296mg

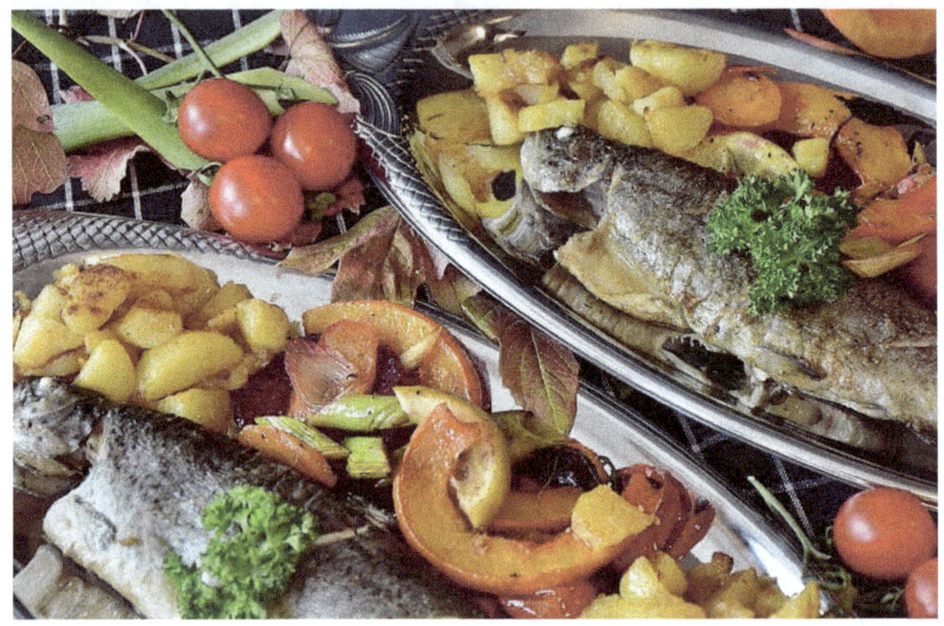

Hot Crab Dip

Preparation time: 10 minutes

Cooking time: 3 hours

Servings: 2

Ingredients:

1/8 cup grated Parmesan cheese

1/4 package cream cheese, softened

1/8 cup mayonnaise

6 oz crabmeat, drained and flaked

Directions:

In a slow cooker, combine the **Ingredients**. Add sweetener to taste and a sliced clove of garlic.

Stir, cover, and cook on low for 2-3 hours .

Nutrition:

Calories: 190 Fat: 16g

Carbs: 3g

Protein: 8g

Cholesterol: 55mg

Sodium: 231mg

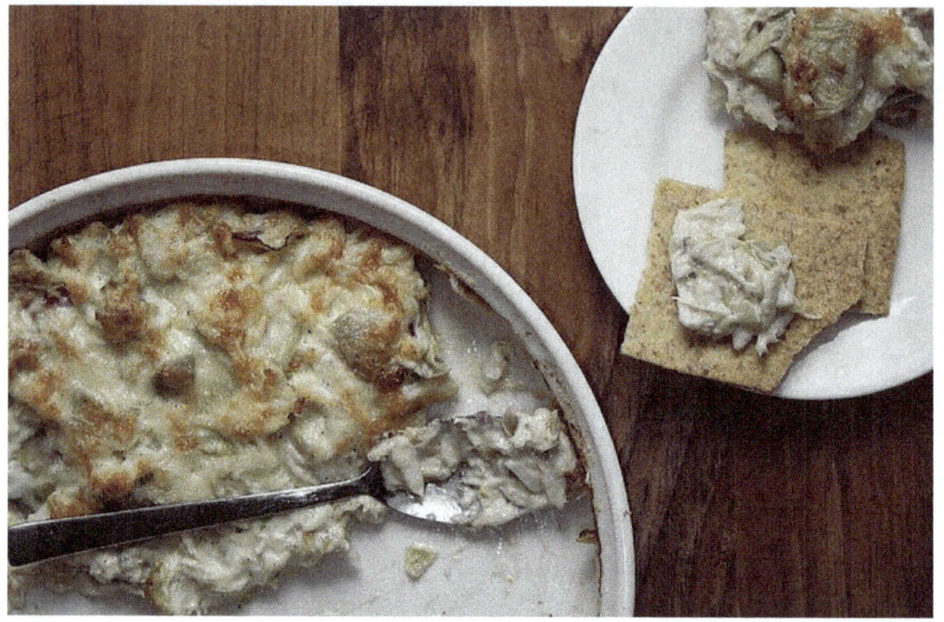

Cod and Zoodles Stew

Preparation time: 5 minutes

Cooking time: 2 hours

Servings: 2

Ingredients:

1/8 cup low-sodium broth

1/2 bell pepper, diced

1/2 lb. sablefish or any whitefish

14 oz diced tomatoes

1 zucchini, made into zoodles

Directions:

Prepare seasonings: onion, garlic, pepper, and salt to taste.

Place all the **Ingredients** in the crockpot and add the prepared seasonings—cook on high for 2 hours.

Nutrition:

Calories: 209 Fat: 20g

Net Carbs: 3g Protein: 15g

Cholesterol: 74mg

Sodium: 291mg

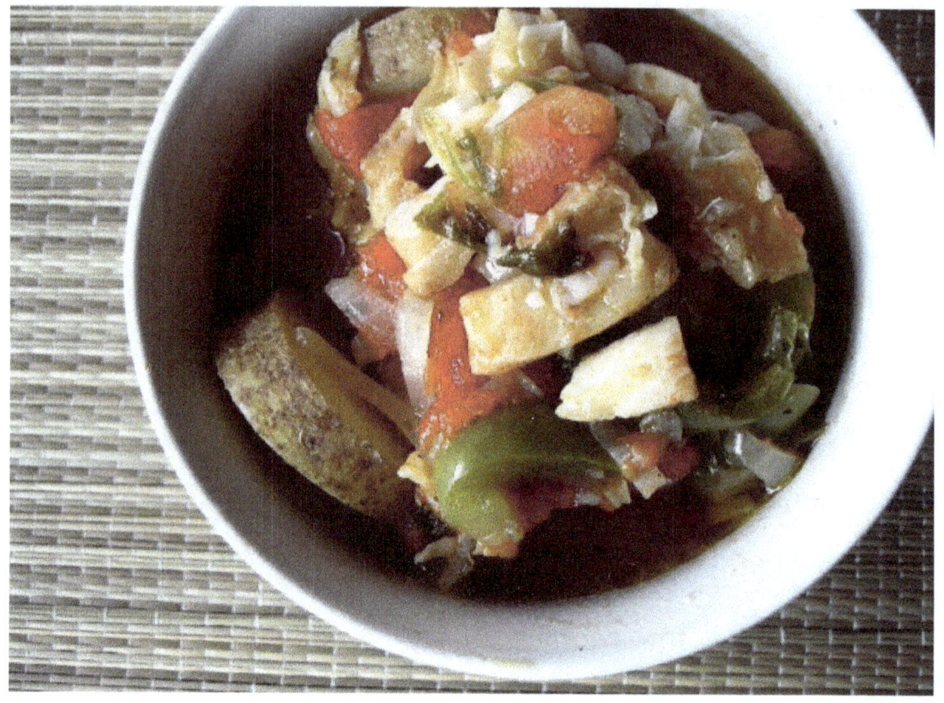

Slow-Cooked Tilapia

Preparation time: 10 minutes

Cooking time: 4 hours

Servings: 2

Ingredients:

1 lb. tilapia, sliced

1/2 fresh lemon, juiced

1/2 cup mayonnaise

Directions:

Whisk mayo and lemon juice in a bowl. Add some chops of garlic.

Spread the mixture on all sides of the tilapia. Cook on low for 3-4 hours.

Nutrition:

Calories: 189 Fat: 18g Carbs: 4g Protein: 22g

Salmon Lemon and Dill

Preparation time: 10 minutes

Cooking time: 2 hours

Servings: 2

Ingredients:

1 tsp extra-virgin olive oil

2 lb. salmon

1 lemon, sliced

A handful of fresh dill

Directions:

Rub salmon with the oil, salt, pepper, garlic, and fresh dill. Put the salmon in the crockpot and place lemon slices on top. Cook on high for 1 hour or low for 2.

Nutrition:

Calories: 159 Fat: 16g Carbs: 2g

Protein: 37g Cholesterol: 114mg

Sodium: 209mg

Creamy Crab Zucchini Casserole

Preparation time: 20 minutes

Cooking time: 5 hours

Servings: 2

Ingredients:

1/4 cup heavy cream

1 medium zucchini squash

2 oz. cream cheese

4 oz. crab meat

1/3 tbsp butter

Directions:

Spiralize zucchini squash on wide ribbons and season with salt. Place the ribbons in a steamer basket and heat for 5 to 7 minutes.

Put all **Ingredients** in a slow cooker, including seasonings such as garlic, onions, pepper, and salt to taste. Put the zucchini spirals on top—Cook within 5 hours on low.

Nutrition: Sodium: 209mg

Calories: 162.6 Fat: 11.9g Carbs: 2.8g

Protein: 7.2g Cholesterol: 114mg

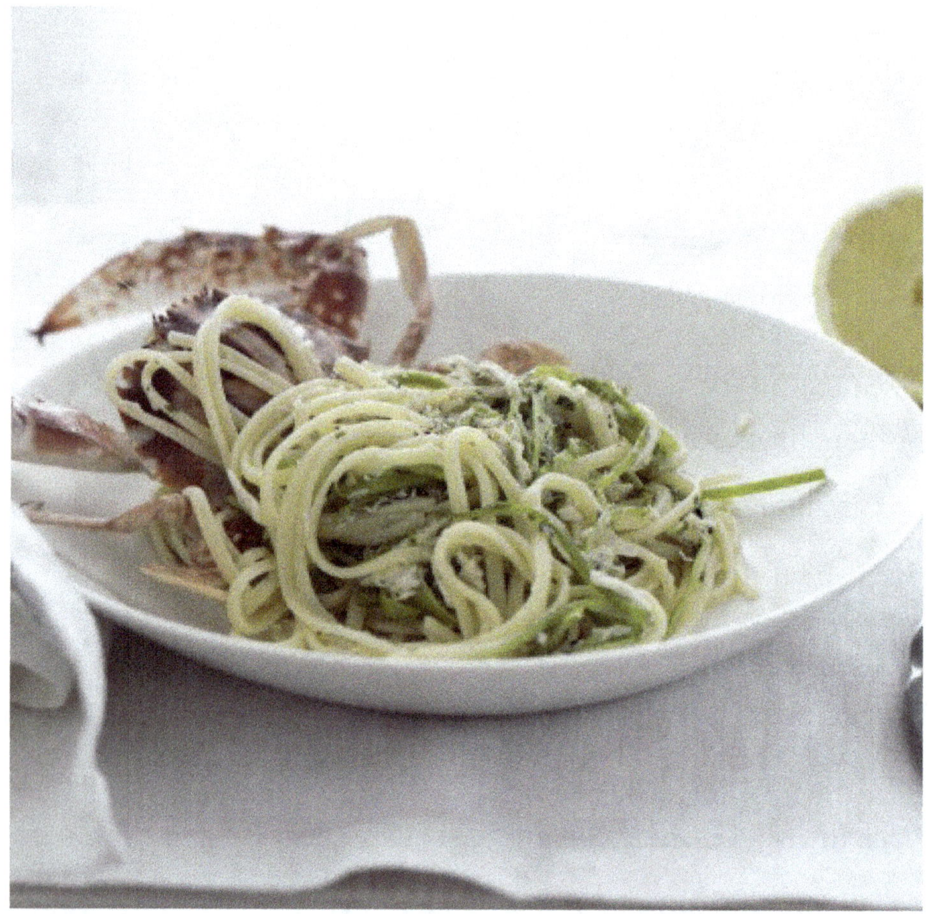

Lobster Bisque

Preparation time: 20 minutes

Cooking time: 6 hours

Servings: 2

Ingredients:

1 1/3 lobster tails, fan parts cut out

2/3 tsp Worcestershire sauce

2 tbsp tomato paste

2/3 cup lobster stock

2/3 cup heavy cream

Directions:

Enhance the broth: slowly add broth to an onion-garlic sauté. Put the broth plus all the other listed fixing except the heavy cream in the crockpot, including desired spices to taste (paprika, thyme, black pepper)—Cook within 6 hours on low.

Nutrition:

Calories: 400 Fat: 30g Carbs: 7g Protein: 23g

Cholesterol: 163mg Sodium: 1758mg

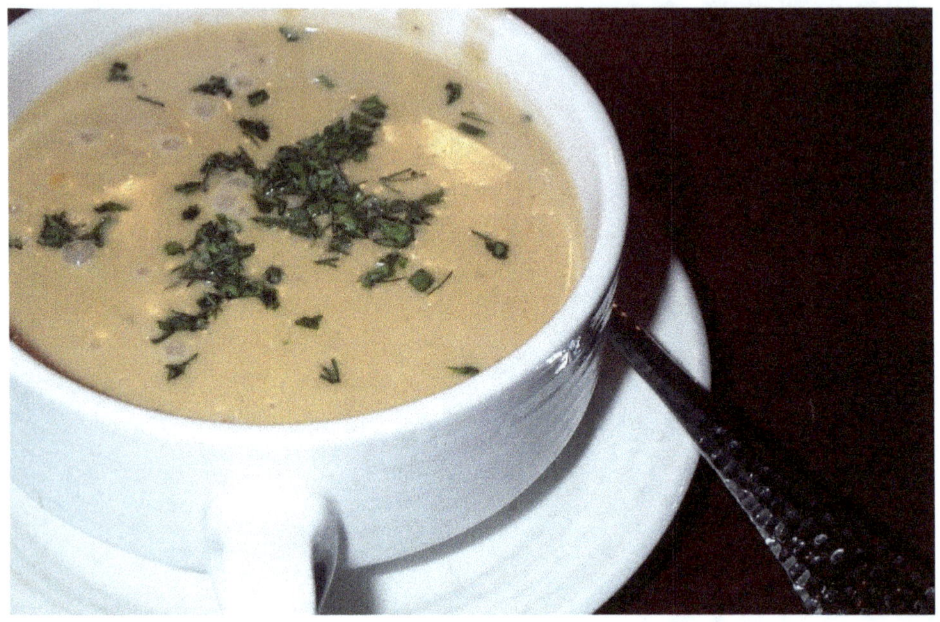

Spicy Shrimp Fra Diavolo

Preparation time: 10 minutes

Cooking time: 3 hours

Servings: 2

Ingredients:

1 teaspoon olive oil

1 onion, diced

5 cloves of garlic, minced

1 teaspoon red pepper flakes

1 can fire-roasted tomatoes

½ teaspoon black pepper

salt to tast e

¼ pound shrimp, shelled and deveined

1 tablespoon Italian parsley

Directions:

Set the crockpot to high heat and heat the oil. Sauté the onion and garlic for 2 minutes.

Add the pepper flakes and tomatoes—season with black pepper and salt.

Add the shrimps. Adjust the heat setting to low and cook for 2 or 3 hours.

Garnish with parsley.

Nutrition:

Calories: 134

Carbohydrates: 3.41 g

Protein: 13.99g

Fat: 3.44 g

Sugar: 1.5g

Sodium: 609mg

Fiber: 0.4g

Shrimp Scampi with Spaghetti Squash

Preparation time: 10 minutes

Cooking time: 2 hours and 20 minutes

Servings: 4

Ingredients:

1 cup broth

2 teaspoon lemon-garlic seasoning

1 onion, chopped

1 tablespoon butter

3 pounds spaghetti squash, cut lengthwise and seeds removed

¾-pounds shrimp, shelled and deveined

Directions:

Pour broth in the slow cooker and add the lemon-garlic seasoning, onion, and butter. Place the spaghetti squash inside the slow cooker and cook on high for 2 hours until soft.

Add the shrimps and cook for 20 more minutes on high.

Nutrition:

Calories: 239

Carbohydrates: 16.79g

Protein: 21.19g

Fat: 6.28g

Sugar: 6.63g

Sodium: 1016mg

Fiber: 5.6g

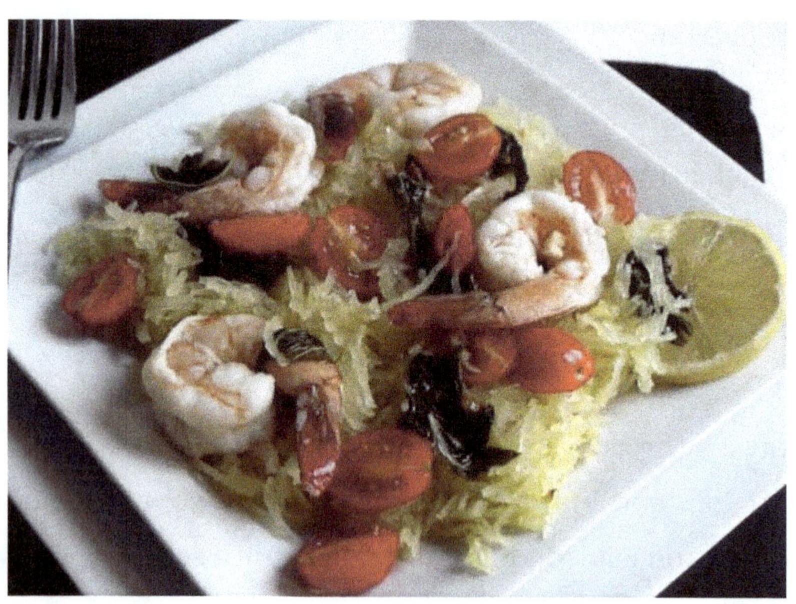

Tuna and White Beans

Preparation time: 10 minutes

Cooking time: 5 hours and 15 minutes

Servings: 4

Ingredients:

4 tablespoon olive oil

1 clove of garlic, minced

6 cups of water

1-pound white beans, soaked overnight and drained

2 cups chopped tomatoes

3 cans white tuna, drained and flaked

2 sprigs of basil

salt and pepper to taste

Directions:

Set the crockpot to high heat and add oil. Sauté the garlic for 2 minutes and add water.

Stir in the beans—Cook within 5 hours on low.

Add in the tomatoes, tuna, and basil—season with salt and pepper to taste.

Continue cooking on high for 15 minutes.

Nutrition:

Calories: 764 Carbohydrates: 12.05g

Protein: 62.84g Fat: 25.43g

Sugar:4 g

Sodium: 559mg

Fiber: 6.03g

Crockpot Swordfish Steaks

Preparation time: 10 minutes

Cooking time: 2 hours

Servings: 6

Ingredients:

6 swordfish steaks

½ cup olive oil

¼ cup lemon juice

½ teaspoon Worcestershire sauce

¼ teaspoon black pepper

1 teaspoon cayenne pepper powder

¼ teaspoon paprika

Directions:

Place the swordfish steaks in the crockpot. Pour the other **Ingredients** over the swordfish steaks.

Close the lid and cook on high for 2 hours. Serve.

Nutrition:

Calories: 659

Carbohydrates: 1.63g

Protein: 46.59g

Fat: 50.78g

Sugar: 0.7g

Sodium: 113mg

Fiber: 0.2g

Sweet and Sour Shrimp

Preparation time: 10 minutes

Cooking time: 5 hours

Servings: 3

Ingredients:

1 package Chinese pea pods, cleaned and trimmed

1 can pineapple tidbits

½ teaspoon ginger, ground

½ pounds shrimps, shelled and deveined

1 cup chicken broth

½ cup pineapple juice

2 tablespoon apple cider vinegar

salt to taste

Directions:

Put the peas in the bottom of the crockpot. Add the pineapple tidbits and ginger.

Place the shrimps on top. Add the chicken broth, pineapple juice, and apple cider vinegar.

Season with salt. Cook on low for 5 hours.

Nutrition:

Calories: 236

Carbohydrates: 3.5 g

Protein: 17.12 g

Fat: 1.33 g Sugar: 1.5g

Sodium: 970 mg

Fiber:0.6 g

Lazy Man's Seafood Stew

Preparation time: 10 minutes

Cooking time: 3 hours

Servings: 6

Ingredients:

1-pound large shrimp

1-pound scallops

1 can crushed tomatoes

4 cloves of garlic, minced

1 tablespoon tomato paste

4 cups vegetable broth

1 teaspoon dried oregano

½ cup onion, chopped

½ teaspoon celery salt

1 teaspoon dried thyme

1/8 teaspoon cayenne pepper

¼ teaspoon red pepper flakes

2 teaspoons salt

2 teaspoons pepper

Directions:

Put all the listed items in the crockpot, then stir to combine.

Close the lid and cook on high for 3 hours or 30 minutes on high setting.

Nutrition:

Calories: 135 Carbohydrates: 9.26g

Protein: 20.37g Fat: 1.29g

Sugar: 3.76g Sodium: 1906mg Fiber:1.3g

Halibut Vinaigrette

Preparation time: 15 minutes

Cooking time: 3 hours

Servings: 6

Ingredients:

2 tablespoon fresh lime juice

1 tablespoon fresh thyme

½ teaspoon crushed red pepper

salt and pepper to taste

4 fillets of halibut fish

1 bunch kale, torn

1 cup of water

1 shallot, sliced

Directions:

Mix lime juice, thyme, red pepper, salt, and pepper. Sprinkle the spices on the halibut fillet.

Place the kale in the crockpot and place the halibut fillet at the bottom. Pour in water and sprinkle shallots on top—Cook within 2 to 3 hours, low.

Nutrition:

Calories: 81

Carbohydrates: 1.25g

Protein: 13.68 g

Fat: 2.12g

Sugar: 0.48g

Sodium: 323mg

Fiber:0.2 g

Crockpot Crab Legs

Preparation time: 10 minutes

Cooking time: 3 hours

Servings: 10

Ingredients:

5 pounds crab legs

1 tablespoon butter

1 teaspoon garlic powder

2 lemons, juiced

salt and pepper to taste

Directions:

Put all **Ingredients** in the pot. Fill the crockpot with ¼ water.

Cook within 3 hours, low. Serve.

Nutrition:

Calories: 294 Carbohydrates: 1.31g

Protein: 49.27g Fat: 8.87g

Sugar: 0.48g Sodium: 175 mg Fiber: 0.1 g

Asian-Inspired Ginger Tuna Steaks

Preparation time: 10 minutes

Cooking time:4 hours

Servings: 2

Ingredients:

2 pounds tuna steak

2 tablespoon coconut aminos

2 tablespoon sherry wine

½ cup of water

6 sprigs of onion, chopped

3 cloves of garlic, minced

1 teaspoon ginger, grated

salt and pepper to taste

Directions:

Place the tuna steak at the bottom of the crockpot.

Add the rest of the **Ingredients**, then marinate.

Cook within 3 to 4 hours, low.

Nutrition:

Calories: 387

Carbohydrates: 12.87g

Protein: 30.65g

Fat: 20.29g

Sugar: 12.9g

Sodium: 91mg

Fiber: 2.4g

Rustic Buttered Mussels

Preparation time: 5 minutes

Cooking time: 3 hours

Servings: 6

Ingredients:

2 pounds mussels, cleaned

½ cup white wine

2 cloves of garlic, minced

1 ¼ tablespoon salt

2 tablespoons butter

Directions:

Place all **Ingredients** in the crockpot.

Cook within 3 hours, low or until the mussels have opened .

Nutrition:

Calories: 167

Carbohydrates: 6.13g

Protein: 18.19g

Fat: 7.23g

Sugar: 0.23g

Sodium: 1918 mg

Fiber:0g

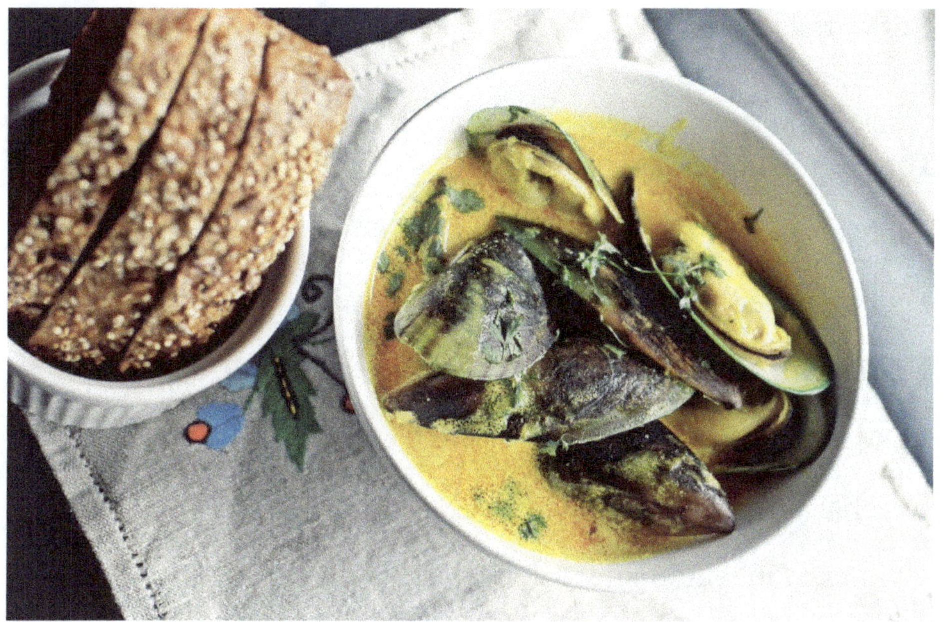

Boiled Lobster Tails

Preparation time: 15 minutes

Cooking time:3 hours

Servings: 4

Ingredients:

4 lobster tails

1 cup of water

4 ounces of white cooking wine

½ stick of butter

½ tablespoon salt

2 tablespoon lemon juice

1 teaspoon rosemary

Directions:

Place all **Ingredients** in the crockpot.

Cook within 3 hours, low or until the lobsters are red.

Nutrition:

Calories: 151

Carbohydrates: 0.56 g

Protein: 30.9g

Fat: 2g

Sugar: 0g

Sodium: 1522mg